TRUE SCARY

CREATURE SIGHTING

HORROR STORIES

TABLE OF CONTENTS:

STORY 1

My name is Tom, and I've been a park ranger at Yosemite National Park for over a decade now. The vast expanse of wilderness, the majestic mountains, and the diverse wildlife have always held a special place in my heart. As a park ranger, it's my duty to protect this natural wonderland and ensure that both the wildlife and visitors are safe.

One crisp morning, as I patrolled my usual route through the dense woods of the park, something caught my attention. A trail of broken branches and disturbed underbrush led me deeper into the forest. Intrigued, I followed the trail, my senses on high alert. As I crept closer, I heard hushed voices and rustling ahead.

Cautiously, I approached and peeked through the thick foliage. What I saw left me dumbfounded. A group of hunters, their faces obscured by camouflage gear, were gathered around a map spread out on the forest floor. They were speaking in low tones, their expressions filled with determination.

My first instinct was to confront them and demand answers. Illegal hunting in the park was not only a violation of the law but also a threat to the delicate balance of the ecosystem. As I stepped into the clearing, the hunters froze, their eyes widening in surprise.

"Who are you?" one of them demanded, trying to mask his unease.

"I'm Tom, a park ranger. What are you doing here, and what are you hunting?" I asked sternly, my gaze flickering between the map and their equipment.

The hunters exchanged uneasy glances before one of them reluctantly spoke up. "We're tracking Bigfoot," he admitted, his voice barely above a whisper.

I couldn't believe what I was hearing. Bigfoot? The mythical creature that had captured the imagination of people for centuries? I had heard rumors and tales, but to think that these hunters were actually pursuing it seemed absurd.

"Hunting any creature in this park is strictly forbidden, especially something as mythical as Bigfoot," I warned, trying to maintain my composure. "You need to pack up and leave immediately."

The hunters hesitated, their expressions conflicted. They were torn between their greed for the supposed fortune that capturing Bigfoot would bring and the fear of facing legal consequences.

I decided to take a different approach. "Listen, I understand your excitement, but chasing after Bigfoot will only lead to trouble. Trust me, I've seen strange things in these woods, and some mysteries are better left unsolved."

Surprisingly, my words seemed to resonate with them, and they began gathering their gear, albeit reluctantly. As they started to leave, I warned them once more about the consequences of their actions and made them promise never to return for such purposes.

For the next few days, I kept a close eye on the area, making sure the hunters didn't return or cause any further trouble. However, they were crafty and managed to evade my surveillance, moving swiftly and leaving no trace behind.

Then, one morning, I noticed something peculiar. The hunters' camp was abandoned, with no sign of their presence. It was as if they had vanished into thin air. I searched the surrounding area, hoping to find clues or any trace of their whereabouts, but it was futile.

Rumors began to spread among the locals and even some visitors about the disappearance of the Bigfoot hunters. Some speculated that they had stumbled upon the elusive creature and met a mysterious fate. Others dismissed it as a wild hoax or a ploy to gain attention.

As for me, I couldn't shake off the feeling of unease. The woods held many secrets, and the disappearance of the hunters only added to the enigma surrounding Yosemite National Park. Whether they had encountered Bigfoot or simply vanished into the wilderness, it remained a mystery that would haunt me for years to come.

STORY 2

The woods have always been my sanctuary, a place where I felt at peace and in tune with nature. As a park ranger, I had spent countless hours exploring every nook and cranny of Yosemite National Park, believing I had seen everything it had to offer. Little did I know that my perception of the wilderness would be forever altered by a chance discovery.

It was a crisp autumn morning when I stumbled upon the artifact. I was on one of my routine patrols, weaving through the dense foliage, when a glint of sunlight caught my eye. Intrigued, I followed the light until I reached a secluded spot where the artifact lay buried beneath a mound of leaves and twigs.

Curiosity piqued, I knelt down and unearthed it with my bare hands. The artifact was unlike anything I had ever seen before. It was a small device adorned with intricate buttons and knobs, its surface shimmering with an otherworldly glow. Despite my lack of knowledge about its origin or purpose, I felt an inexplicable pull towards it.

As I held the artifact in my hands, a strange sensation washed over me. It was as if the device was alive, pulsating with an energy that seemed to attract something unseen yet undeniably dangerous. At first, I dismissed it as a figment of my imagination, a trick of the mind brought on by the artifact's mysterious allure.

But as I continued my patrol through the woods, the feeling of being watched intensified. Every rustle of leaves, every snap of a twig sent shivers down my spine. It was as if a predator lurked just beyond my line of sight, stalking me with deadly intent.

Then it struck, swift and silent. The predator was like a shadow, blending seamlessly with the surroundings. Its movements were fluid and precise, its sharp claws and teeth gleaming in the dappled sunlight. I barely had time to react before it pounced, forcing me into a desperate struggle for survival.

My training as a ranger kicked in, and I reached for my gun, hoping to fend off the creature. But my weapon proved futile against its speed and agility. It was clear that I was outmatched, facing a foe unlike any I had encountered before.

To my astonishment, the predator seemed fixated on the artifact in my possession. It snarled and lunged, driven by an insatiable desire to reclaim what it believed to be its own. I realized then that the artifact held a power that drew the creature to it, a power I couldn't comprehend.

With adrenaline coursing through my veins, I made a split-second decision. I activated the artifact, and to my amazement, it emitted a blinding light that repelled the predator. Seizing the opportunity, I sprinted through the woods, the creature's enraged cries fading behind me.

When I finally reached the safety of the ranger station, I was shaken and bewildered. I knew I had narrowly escaped a deadly encounter, but the mystery surrounding the artifact and the creature left me with more questions than answers.

I made the decision to lock away the artifact in a secure location within the station, knowing that its power posed a grave danger if it fell into the wrong hands. But even as I secured it, I couldn't shake the feeling that the woods held secrets far beyond our understanding.

Days turned into weeks, and yet the memory of that encounter lingered, haunting me like a specter. I could still feel the predator's presence, a constant reminder of the unknown lurking in the depths of the forest.

As I continued my duties as a park ranger, I couldn't help but wonder about the artifact's origins and the creature it had attracted. Were there more of its kind out there, hidden from human eyes? Or was it a unique anomaly, a chance convergence of worlds?

One thing was certain - the woods held mysteries beyond imagination, and my encounter with the artifact and the predator was just a glimpse into a realm of possibilities I could barely fathom. And as I gazed out into the wilderness, I knew that my journey as a park ranger was far from over, filled with untold adventures and dangers waiting to be uncovered.

STORY 3

As a 27-year-old guy living in the western part of Norway, I've always had a deep love for the outdoors. Whether it's fishing, jogging, playing sports, or hiking, I find solace and joy in nature's embrace. However, one particular camping trip in the woods left me with an experience I'll never forget and a newfound fear that still lingers in my mind.

It was a typical Saturday afternoon when I decided to embark on a solo camping trip to a local mountain. Being 194 centimeters tall (or 6 feet 4 inches in U.S. measurements) and weighing 230 pounds, I considered myself fairly athletic and not easily scared. Little did I know that this trip would test my courage in ways I never imagined.

The hike to the camping spot was steep but manageable. After a few hours of trekking, I reached a beautiful clearing and set up my tent. The Norwegian evening was clear and serene, typical of summer weather in the region. I started a fire, cooked some food, and enjoyed the peaceful ambiance of the forest.

As the sun began to set, I felt a sense of relaxation wash over me. I planned to unwind with a book by the fire, but the darkness made it challenging to read. That's when I heard a noise coming from a nearby bush. At first, I dismissed it as a small animal rustling around. But then, I saw it.

Standing to my right and slightly ahead was a creature unlike anything I had ever encountered. It wasn't the massive 7 to 9-foot monster described in reports, but it was still intimidating. It stood about 6 feet tall and emitted heavy, animal-like breaths that sent a shiver down my spine.

Frozen in fear, I sat motionless as the creature stared at me. Its dark eyes were shadowed by brow ridges, making it impossible to discern its intentions. I couldn't move or speak; I was afraid of provoking it further.

The creature's movements were slow and deliberate, reminiscent of a cat stalking its prey. Every inch it inched closer, my heart raced faster. Without thinking, I grabbed a handful of red glowing sticks from the fire and hurled them towards the creature.

The sudden burst of light and heat startled the creature, causing it to bolt into the darkness. I sat there, trembling and trying to process what had just happened. It felt like an eternity, even though the encounter lasted mere moments.

To this day, I haven't been back to that part of the woods. The fear of the unknown and the encounter with that creature have kept me away. I've shared my story with a few close friends and family members, but it's not something I openly discuss.

I often wonder what that creature was and if anyone else has encountered something similar. Was it a rare animal or something supernatural? I may never know the truth, but that night in the woods will always remain etched in my memory as a chilling reminder of the mysteries that lurk in the wilderness.

STORY 4

The month-long camping trip with my boyfriend, Jason, had been an adventure filled with memorable experiences and breathtaking landscapes. However, everything took a chilling turn on October 9th when we decided to deviate from our planned campground reservation and opt for a spontaneous camping spot near Albion Basin in the Uinta Mountains of Alta, Utah.

The decision to try dispersed camping for the first time was met with a mix of excitement and apprehension. We lacked proper backpacking gear but were determined to make the most of our impromptu camping escapade. Little did we know that this decision would lead us into a night of terror we would never forget.

Arriving at Albion Basin Campground around 3 PM, we realized that the area we wanted to camp in was a strenuous 2-mile uphill hike. Initially, we expressed regret for skipping our planned campsite in Nephi, Utah, but our adventurous spirits pushed us forward. After a hearty lunch to avoid carrying excess food, we packed our backpacks with the best gear we had and set out on the trail, hoping to find a suitable spot for the night.

As we trudged along, the weight of our decision began to sink in. We questioned why we had chosen this path, feeling a sense of unease creeping over us. Despite these feelings, we pressed on, fueled by a desire to prove ourselves and embrace the challenge.

Upon reaching Cecret Lake, we found it disappointingly empty and eerie, not at all like the picturesque images we had seen. Undeterred, we continued hiking in search of seclusion and a flat camping spot. That's when I spotted a small cave in the distance, prompting us to debate whether it was safe to camp nearby. Jason investigated and deemed it a harmless animal crawl space, easing our concerns.

Nightfall descended quickly, and we set up camp, playing cards and enjoying the warmth of the fire. However, as the hours passed and we settled in for bed around 8:30 PM, an inexplicable sense of dread began to creep over me.

At 11:24 PM, I woke up abruptly, feeling a deep sense of fear unlike anything I had experienced before. I lay awake, alert, and unnerved, unable to shake the feeling of impending danger. Jason was asleep beside me, unaware of my turmoil.

Around midnight, Jason stirred awake, providing some comfort as I struggled with my fear. He suggested I try to rest, but neither of us could find peace. Eventually, I confessed my fear, and we decided to tough it out until morning, relying on the small axe and pellet gun for protection.

Minutes later, as we lay wide awake, Jason's sudden alertness startled me. He gestured for me to listen, and in the eerie silence of the night, we heard the unmistakable sound of gravel crunching under footsteps outside our tent. Fear gripped us both as the footsteps approached and stopped near my side of the tent.

My heart raced as Jason grabbed the gun and rushed outside, ready to confront whoever or whatever was there. But to our shock, there was nothing. The footsteps had ceased abruptly, leaving us with a sense of dread and confusion.

Packing up hastily, we descended the mountain in the moonlit darkness, too afraid to use our flashlights. The fear of being watched and followed haunted us as we made it back to our car around 3:30 AM, seeking refuge in a well-lit grocery store parking lot to catch some much-needed sleep.

Since that night, Jason and I have discussed our harrowing experience countless times, haunted by the memory of those inexplicable footsteps and the chilling feeling of being watched in the wilderness. It's a night we'll never forget, a reminder of the unknown dangers that lurk in the depths of nature.

STORY 5

As a park ranger in Northern Minnesota's Voyageurs National Park, I had experienced my fair share of wildlife encounters. From bears to wolves and moose, I thought I had seen and heard it all. However, one fateful night changed everything and left me haunted for years to come.

It was a serene and beautiful evening, calm and warm, the kind of night that makes you appreciate the wonders of nature. After a long day of work, I sat on a dock with a co-worker, gazing up at the starry sky and engaging in deep conversations about life. That's when it happened—a howl unlike anything I had ever heard before echoed through the woods.

The sound was distorted, powerful, and seemed to emanate from something with massive lungs. It lasted an astonishing 18 seconds, starting low in pitch and ending with a higher tone. It was a continuous howl with no breaks or pauses, and it felt like it was coming from the south, very close to where we were.

Without hesitation, we ran inside to grab our guns and lights, determined to investigate the source of the eerie howl. Venturing into the woods, we heard the howl again, this time from the east. Undeterred, we returned to our camping trailer, retrieved our recording equipment, and headed back into the woods to capture the mysterious sound.

Setting up the microphones, we recorded the howl a total of four times. Upon playing back the recordings in our office, we noticed something unsettling. In the background of the howl, there was a loud growling sound that seemed to grow closer as the howl progressed. It was as if whatever was making the howl was approaching us.

What was even more chilling was the response we captured—a distinct howl from the other side of the lake, a call and response between two large creatures. Despite being barely audible in the recording, it was clear that something significant was happening in the woods that night.

Excited by our findings, we were ready to share our discovery, but our supervisor shut down the entire investigation immediately. His seriousness and anger were palpable as he warned us never to speak of the incident again, threatening us with termination if we did.

Fearing for our jobs, we complied with his orders and destroyed the tapes, erasing any evidence of the strange howls and growls. However, the memory of that night has haunted me for the past 15 years. I've tried to bury the experience and distract myself with other matters, but it always lingers in the back of my mind.

I know there is something out there, something large, powerful, and not natural. It's a feeling that gnaws at me, leaving me curious yet terrified of what lurks in the depths of the woods. As a ranger, I pride myself on knowing the wildlife in my area, but whatever made those sounds remains a mystery to this day.

That's why I reached out to you. I needed someone to talk to, someone who would take me seriously and listen without judgment. I cannot risk revealing my identity, as it could cost me my job and reputation with the U.S. National Park Service. Please keep my name confidential and thank you for lending an ear to my unsettling experience.

STORY 6

The most unbelievable threats can be overcome with courage and unity. However, my journey through Willowbrook was far from over. The echoes of that harrowing experience continued to linger in my mind, prompting me to delve deeper into the mysteries surrounding the town and the creature that had plagued it.

Despite the victory over the malevolent force, questions remained unanswered. What was the origin of the creature? How did it come to be? And most importantly, were there more of its kind out there, lurking in the shadows of other towns?

My curiosity and determination drove me to seek answers, leading me down a path filled with research and investigation. I spent countless hours pouring over old folklore, legends, and historical records, trying to piece together the puzzle of Willowbrook's dark past.

As I delved deeper into the town's history, I uncovered tales of ancient rituals, whispered incantations, and a dark pact made with an otherworldly entity. It seemed that Willowbrook had always been a nexus of supernatural activity, hidden beneath a facade of quaint small-town life.

Armed with newfound knowledge, I sought out experts in the occult and paranormal, hoping to gain insight into the creature's true nature. Together, we pieced together fragments of information, painting a picture of a being born from forbidden magic and bound by an insatiable hunger for souls.

But the more I learned, the more I realized that Willowbrook was just one piece of a much larger puzzle. Similar incidents had occurred in neighboring towns, each with its own tale of terror and inexplicable disappearances. It was as if a web of darkness stretched across the region, connecting these isolated incidents into a sinister pattern.

Determined to break this cycle of fear and suffering, I joined forces with other investigators, forming a network dedicated to uncovering the truth behind these supernatural occurrences. We shared our findings, pooled our resources, and devised strategies to confront the hidden threats lurking in the shadows.

Our efforts led us to confrontations with entities beyond human comprehension—ancient spirits, demonic entities, and creatures born from nightmares. Each encounter tested our courage and resolve, pushing us to the brink of our capabilities.

But through sheer determination and unwavering unity, we managed to thwart these dark forces time and again. Slowly but surely, we chipped away at the web of darkness that had ensnared our region for centuries.

Years passed, and our efforts bore fruit as the incidents of supernatural activity dwindled, and towns once shrouded in fear found peace once more. Willowbrook, once a hotbed of terror, became a symbol of resilience and triumph over adversity.

As I reflect on those turbulent times, I am reminded of the power of unity and perseverance. Together, we faced the unknown, confronted our fears, and emerged stronger than ever. And while the memories of those dark days may never fade entirely, they serve as a reminder of the indomitable human spirit and our ability to overcome even the most daunting challenges.

STORY 7

I had been a park ranger for more than a decade, patrolling the vast and remote national park that was both my workplace and my sanctuary. It was a typical day like any other when the distress call came in—a group of experienced hikers had gone missing, and my instincts told me that something was terribly wrong.

Without hesitation, I geared up and set out to find them. The forest was dense, and navigating through the thick underbrush was no easy task. As I ventured deeper into the woods, a sense of unease began to creep over me. It was as if the very trees were whispering warnings, urging me to turn back.

Ignoring the ominous feeling, I pressed on, determined to locate the missing hikers. The rustling of leaves and the occasional snap of a twig made me acutely aware that I was not alone. Every fiber of my being screamed danger, but I pushed forward, driven by a sense of duty and urgency.

Hours passed as I followed what little evidence I could find—a broken branch here, a discarded piece of equipment there. It wasn't long before I stumbled upon a makeshift campsite, and my heart sank. Tents were torn open, belongings scattered, and there was no sign of the hikers.

As I surveyed the scene, a primal growl echoed through the trees, sending a chill down my spine. I drew my weapon, scanning the area for any sign of movement. That's when I saw it—an enormous creature emerging from the shadows.

It stood tall and imposing, with matted fur and claws that glinted in the dim light. My training kicked in, and I aimed my weapon, ready to defend myself. But this creature was unlike anything I had ever encountered. It was intelligent, calculating, and clearly hunting me.

I fired a warning shot, hoping to scare it off, but it only seemed to anger the creature. It charged towards me with lightning speed, and I knew I had to run. Adrenaline surged through my veins as I sprinted through the dense forest, the creature hot on my heels.

I could feel its breath on my neck, its claws scraping against my skin. Panic threatened to overwhelm me, but I pushed through, driven by sheer survival instinct. Just when I thought I couldn't run any longer, I stumbled and fell.

I braced myself for the inevitable attack, but to my surprise, the creature stopped abruptly. It looked up towards the sky, emitting a deafening roar before vanishing back into the depths of the forest. I was left shaken and bewildered, but alive.

Regaining my composure, I continued my search for the missing hikers. It took hours of scouring the area, but eventually, I found them—traumatized but alive. They recounted tales of a monstrous creature stalking them, confirming my own encounter.

I ensured they received the medical attention they needed and escorted them back to safety. But the memory of that creature lingered, haunting my thoughts day and night. What was it? Where did it come from? And why did it spare me in the end?

The woods held secrets beyond comprehension, mysteries that may never be unraveled. As a park ranger, I had seen my fair share of darkness, but nothing could have prepared me for the enigma that lurked within those ancient trees.

STORY 8

It was the summer of 2002, and my family and I were on a trip to Oregon to visit my dad in Parkdale, Hood River. Nestled in the midst of forested areas, his place was a serene escape from the hustle and bustle of city life. Little did we know that our tranquil getaway would turn into a series of eerie encounters that would haunt us for years to come.

One night, after a long day of driving, we were all exhausted and settled into our camper for the night. It was around 3 in the morning when my mother, for some inexplicable reason, found herself wide awake. She lay in bed, listening to the soothing sounds of nature when suddenly, chaos erupted outside.

My dad's peacocks, ducks, and guinea hens started squawking and making a ruckus. At first, my mom assumed it was just a fox or some other animal intruding into the hen house. But then, as quickly as it had started, the commotion ceased, leaving an eerie silence in its wake.

That's when my mom heard it—a series of loud, guttural screams and yells coming from not too far away. As she lay there, listening intently, her mind raced through all the animals she knew from her time working in a zoo. None of them matched the unearthly sound she was hearing.

The screaming continued for a few terrifying moments before gradually fading away into the distance. Eventually, exhaustion overtook her, and she drifted off to sleep. It wasn't until the next morning that she recounted the unnerving experience to my sister and me.

As she relayed the events of that night, chills ran down my spine. Memories flooded back to me from a few years prior when I used to visit my dad's place during the summers. I remembered one particular night when my dad's dog, sleeping in a kennel beside me, suddenly started growling and barking ferociously.

At the time, I had brushed it off as just the dog being spooked by a passing animal. But now, with my mom's story fresh in my mind, a new thought crossed my mind—what if it wasn't just any animal outside? What if it was something much more elusive and mysterious?

Just a few nights before my mom heard those spine-chilling screams, my sister and I had a bizarre encounter while driving into Oregon. I was behind the wheel, and my sister was in the passenger seat when we both saw a massive, black figure crossing the road just at the edge of our headlights' reach.

I remember the shock and confusion that swept over us as we passed by, both of us questioning what we had just seen. It was a fleeting moment, but it left an indelible mark on our minds.

When my mom insisted that I pull over and let her take the wheel that night, I hesitated. Fear gnawed at me, not just from the unknown creature we had seen crossing the road, but also from the unnerving screams my mom had heard in the dead of night.

As I handed over the keys to my mom and climbed into the passenger seat, a sense of unease settled over me. What if Bigfoot, or whatever creature roamed these woods, was watching us from the shadows? What if these encounters were more than just coincidences?

To this day, the memory of that summer trip to Oregon lingers in my mind, a testament to the mysterious and unexplained forces that sometimes lurk in the darkness of the wilderness. Whether it was a figment of our imagination or something more tangible, those nights in the woods left an imprint on our souls, forever altering our perception of the natural world.

STORY 9

The events I'm about to recount still send shivers down my spine whenever I think about them. It was a series of encounters with something inexplicable and terrifying, something that defied all logical explanations.

It all started innocently enough, on a lazy summer day at the city park with my friend Mike and two girls we had met recently. We were lounging on the grass, enjoying the warmth of the sun, when we heard it—a deep, guttural sound that seemed to come from the hill behind us. It was unlike anything I had ever heard before, and it sent a chill down my spine.

At first, we dismissed it as some strange echo or maybe a prank by someone nearby. But curiosity got the better of us, and three days later, we found ourselves back at the park, eager to unravel the mystery of that eerie sound.

As we stood at the same spot where we had heard the sound, I noticed something strange. At first, I mistook it for a tall pole, swaying gently in the breeze. But upon closer inspection, I realized there was something more to it. It was like a humanoid figure, wavering in the distance.

I called Mike over to take a look, but by the time he reached me, the figure had vanished into thin air. Confused and slightly unnerved, we scanned the hillside, but there was no sign of anyone or anything. We chalked it up to imagination or maybe a trick of the light and shrugged it off.

However, our peace was short-lived. A few days later, Mike and I decided to visit our family farm, located about three miles away from the city park. It was a routine check-up since nobody lived there, and we wanted to make sure everything was in order.

As we turned into the driveway and the headlights illuminated the area, that's when we saw it again. It was standing right there, near the old fence line, casually stepping over a 5-strand barbed wire fence as if it were nothing. Its proportions were human-like, but its movements were far from ordinary.

The most unsettling part was its eyes—they glowed in the light, reflecting an animal-like intensity. We froze for a moment, trying to process what we were seeing. It was like a scene from a horror movie come to life.

Without exchanging a word, we instinctively knew we had to get out of there, and fast. We reversed the car and sped away from the farm, leaving the creature behind in the darkness.

For weeks after that incident, Mike and I couldn't shake off the feeling of dread and unease. We tried to rationalize what we had seen, coming up with explanations ranging from a misidentified animal to a prank by someone in the area.

But deep down, we knew that what we had encountered defied any logical explanation. It was something otherworldly, something that lurked in the shadows and evoked primal fear.

To this day, we avoid talking about those sightings, fearing that we might attract unwanted attention from whatever that creature was. It remains a chilling mystery, a haunting memory that serves as a stark reminder of the unknown dangers that lurk in the world around us.